Flexitarian Diet

Best And Simple Recipes For Weight Loss, Disease Prevention, And Plant-based Meals

(Feel Incredible Using The Ultimate In Flexible Dieting)

Alícia-Yves Ahmad

TABLE OF CONTENT

Introduction 1

Chapter 1: Possibly Beneficial To The Environment 7

Chapter 2: What Foods Do San Flextaran Consume? 9

Chapter 3: Some Strategies For Transitioning To A Plant-Based Diet 13

Chapter 4: What Are The Meat-Related Guidelines For The Flexitarian Diet? 22

Chapter 5: What Exactly Is A Flexitarian Diet? 25

Chapter 6: A Summary Of Flextaran Det 33

Garlic & Tomato Pasta 40

Shepherd's Pie 43

Chapter 7: Be Beneficial To The Environment 48

Asian-Style Wellington Mushroom 53

Spiralized Zucchini And Smoked Salmon, With A Vegetarian Twist 58

- Vegetable Spring Quiche 61
- Orange Gelatin 64
- Oatmeal & Egg Whites 66
- Spaghetti With Spinach And Lemon With Almonds 68
- Black Bean Tostadas 70
- Vegan Blats 73
- Apple Butter Recipe 75
- Marinated Fajita Chicken 79
- No-Guilt Zesty Ranch Dip 82

Introduction

Flexitarianism is not only a viable option for meat eaters who are attracted to vegetarianism, but also for vegetarians who want to incorporate a small amount of meat into their diet for health reasons or personal preferences. Simply reducing the amount of meat in your diet will not result in a noticeable weight loss unless you are aware of what you are replacing the meat with and easy make a concerted effort to choose the appropriate foods. The best way for flexitarians to replace some of their meat consumption is by consuming more nutritious protein sources. Included among these are:

Eggs; an omelette filled with fresh vegetables is an excellent source of protein that will also leave you feeling satisfied and satiated.

Meat substitutes such as tofu, Quorn, and soya are utilised in an assortment of inventive ways.

Try substituting kidney beans, lentils, and chickpeas for ground beef in chilli con carne made with legumes (beans, peas, and pulses).

Nuts and seeds; occasionally snacking on nuts and seeds is an excellent way to consume healthy fats and protein.

This book, Flexitarian Diet Easy cook book for Beginners, will teach you everything you need to know about the Flexitarian Diet and provide you with 82 easy-to-easy make recipes to help you along your flexitarian journey.

Weight management

Flexitarian eating may also aid in weight management.

This is partially due to the fact that flexitarians typically consume fewer high-calorie, highly processed foods and more naturally low-calorie plant foods.

Multiple studies have demonstrated that people who adhere to a plant-based diet tend to lose more weight than those who do not.

Those who consumed a vegetarian diet for 2 8 weeks gained 8 .10 pounds (2 kilogrammes) more than those who did not, according to a review of studies involving over 2 ,2 00 people.

Vegans are more likely to be overweight than vegetarians and omnivores, according to this and other studies.

Because the Flexitarian Diet is more similar to a vegetarian diet than a vegan diet, it may aid in weight loss, but perhaps not as much as a vegan diet would.

However, weight loss is not the main objective of the Flextaran Diet. It is more focused on incorporating more nutrient-dense foods, such as fruits, legumes, and vegetables, into your diet.

Diabetes type 2 is a global health crisis. A healthy diet, particularly one based on rredomnantlu rlants, may help prevent and manage this disease. This is likely due to the fact that plant-based diets promote weight loss and contain numerous foods that are high in fibre and low in unhealthy fats and added sugar. A study with over 200,000 participants found that a diet high in plant foods and low in animal foods was associated with a 20% lower risk of developing diabetes.

In addition, a diet that emphasised healthy plant foods was associated with a 6 8 % reduction in diabetes risk, whereas a diet high in less healthy plant foods was associated with a 2 6% increase in diabetes risk. The healthy plant-based diet included whole grains, fruits, vegetables, nuts, legumes, and vegetable oil, while the less healthy plant-based diet included fruit juices, sweetened beverages, refined grains, and sweets.

The reduction in HbA2 s (6 -month average of blood sugar readings) was greater in people with plant-based diets than in those with conventional diets, according to additional research.

Detaru rattern high in nutrient-dense plant foods, such as fruits, vegetables, and legumes, and low in ultra-refined foods are associated with a reduced risk of developing certain diseases. Vegetarian diets are associated with a lower incidence of all cancers, but especially soloretal cancers, according to research. A 7-year study of sae of colorectal cancers in 78,000 reorle revealed that semi-vegetarians were 8% less likely to develop this type of cancer than non-vegetarians.

Therefore, incorporating more vegetarian foods by consuming a flexitarian diet may reduce your risk of developing cancer.

The Flexitarian Diet may aid in weight management and lower the risk of cardiovascular disease, cancer, and type 2 diabetes. Due to the fact that most research examines vegetarian and vegan diets, it is difficult to determine whether flexitarian eating has comparable health benefits.

Chapter 1: Possibly Beneficial To The Environment

The Flexitarian Diet may provide health and environmental benefits. Reducing meat consumption can aid in preserving natural resources by reducing greenhouse gas emissions and land and water consumption. A review of the research on the sustainability of plant-based diets revealed that switching from the typical Western diet to a flexitarian one, in which meat is rarely replaced by plant foods, could reduce greenhouse gas emissions by 7%.

Eating more rlant foods will also increase the demand for more land to be devoted to growing fruits and vegetables for humans rather than animal feed. Rlant cultivation requires significantly fewer resources than animal husbandry.

In fact, greenhoue gas emissions resulting from vegan and ovo-lasto-vegetaran diets are approximately 10 0 and 6 10 percent lower, respectively, than those from the majority of current omnvore diets, with corresponding reductions in the use of natural resources. Diets based on plants require fewer fossil fuels and less land and water.

Chapter 2: What Foods Do San Flextaran Consume?

"All food grains are included in the diet," said Blatner. "with the exception that there is less emphasis on anmal rroten and more on rlant-rroten." Blatner recommends centering uour meal around plant-proteins, lke black bean, pinto bean, garbanzo bean, and lentl, sourled wth whole grains and potatoes, vegetable, frut, dairy, egg, and health fat, lke olve oil, avoado oil, and fh.

Since the Flexitarian Diet actively seeks to reduce meat consumption, the meal plan will consist primarily of plant-based foods.

Options for plant-based foods on the flexitarian diet include:

Whole grains. Whole grain examples would include rye, oats, barley, and buckwheat. Most grain-based diets contain a substantial amount of whole grains.

Vegetables. Obviously, even semi-vegetarian diets will contain a great deal of vegetables! And they should be because vegetables are healthy. They are packed with nutrients, fibre, and are typically low in calories. Most reorle could benefit from eating more vegetables. If you are unable to stomach greens, I've got you covered. Check out the passage for advice on how to convert any vegetable-hater.

Legumes. Beans, lentils, and sou easy make ur the legume familu. When eliminating meat, legumes are an excellent source of protein (more on this below).

Fruit. Since bananas, apples, and oranges all originate from plants, they are all vegetarian-friendly. While they are high in sugar, they are also nutrient-deficient. Our standard recommendation regarding fruit consumption is to consume whole fruits and avoid fruit juices.

Seeds and nuts. Again, they are derived from plants, so almond, cashew, and pumpkin seeds are appropriate for any vegetable you select. So quinoa, which is commonly regarded as a grain, is actually a seed. Mind=blown. Although high in fat and calories, nuts and seeds are another excellent source of protein in a semi-vegetarian diet.

Chapter 3: Some Strategies For Transitioning To A Plant-Based Diet

Consume many vegetables. Fill a portion of your lunch and dinner plate with vegetables. Ensure you remember a large number of vegetable varieties when picking them. Recognize vegetables as an accompaniment to hummus, salsa, or guacamole.

Change the manner in which you consider meat significantly. Have more modest sums. Use it as a supplement rather than the main focus.

Pick great fats. The fats found in olive oil, olives, nuts and nut butters, seeds, and avocados are incredibly nutritious.

Easy cook a vegan feast equivalent to one night per week. Organize these meals around legumes, whole grains, and vegetables.

Include whole grains in your breakfast. Start with grain, cereal, quinoa, or buckwheat. Then, add a few nuts or seeds to the fresh produce.

Go for greens. Every day, consume a variety of green vegetables, including kale, collards, Swiss chard, and spinach. Steam, grill, braise, or sauté food to preserve its flavour and nutrients.

Build a meal around a portion of mixed greens. Fill a bowl with salad greens such as romaine lettuce, spinach, Bibb lettuce, and red mixed greens. Add a variety of vegetables along with fresh spices, beans, peas, or tofu.

Consume organic products as dessert. After a meal, a ready, delicious peach, an invigorating slice of watermelon, or a crisp apple will satisfy your sweet tooth.

Moved oats with pecans, banana, and a sprinkle of cinnamon.

Breakfast wrap: Fill an entire wheat tortilla with fried egg, dark beans, peppers, onions, Monterey jack cheddar, and a sprinkle of hot sauce or salsa.Entire wheat English biscuit finished off with new tomato and avocado cuts, and blueberries.

Cleaved mixed greens are tossed with fresh tomato, Kalamata olives, fresh parsley, crumbled feta cheddar, extra virgin olive oil, and balsamic vinegar for a Greek salad. Complete whole wheat pita as an afterthought, fresh melon for dessert.

Apple, tomato basil soup, and whole grain wafers with tabbouleh.

Vegetable lover pizza topped with cheddar mozzarella, tomatoes, broccoli, onions, peppers, and mushrooms. Strawberries for dessert are fresh.

Grilled vegetable skewers served with grilled tofu and a quinoa and spinach salad.

Whole wheat pasta with cannellini beans and peas, accompanied by a romaine salad with cherry tomatoes dressed with extra virgin olive oil and balsamic vinegar.

Vegan bean stew served with a spinach-orzo salad.

Whole plant-based food sources contain a high amount of fibre, no dietary cholesterol, and low amounts of saturated fats — an ideal combination for heart health. Currently, meat, cheese, and eggs contain cholesterol and saturated fats that, when consumed in excess, can promote plaque formation in a person's arteries.

However, it is sufficient not to avoid meat entirely: For heart health on a plant-based diet, it is essential to avoid processed foods like white rice and white bread, which lack nutritional value and have a high glycemic index. This increases the likelihood of glucose spikes and increased cravings. Additionally, whole organic fruits are more wholesome than organic fruit juice, even 2 00 percent juice, which frequently loses vitamins and nutrients during processing and is high in sugar.

Multiple studies have demonstrated the cholesterol-lowering effects of plant-based diets, particularly a veggie lover or vegetarian diet with nuts, soy, and fibre. Five observational studies, cited in a 2009 review published in the American Journal of Cardiology, discovered lower blood concentrations of TC and LDL cholesterol in populations consuming plant-based calories.

Vegetarians and vegetarians who consume fewer calories have been shown to promote a healthy balance of beneficial microorganisms that promote stomach and overall health. A healthy stomach biome promotes an advanced framework for digestion, solid defecation, and adequate levels of chemicals that contribute to adequate hunger regulation.

According to research led by Hana Kahleova, M.D., Ph.D., of the Doctors Council on Dependable Medication and presented at the 202 9 meeting of the European Association for the Study of Diabetes in Barcelona, only 2 6 weeks of a healthy vegetarian diet centred on whole foods grown from the ground has been shown to improve stomach health.

Reduced risk for specific cancers

Plants produce an abundance of phytochemicals that are both protective against cell damage and calming. Different long-term studies suggest that the benefits of consuming whole plant foods as opposed to processed foods may have the potential to prevent up to

6 6 percent of all disease cases. Most research has focused on the protective effects of plant-based diets against breast, colorectal, gastrointestinal, and prostate diseases.

Reduced joint inflammation discomfort

Low-fat, high-fiber diets have been shown to reduce inflammation, which is excellent news for those adhering to a plant-based, whole-foods diet. As a result of how effective plants are at reducing inflammation, plant-based calorie counts have been shown to be beneficial for those with inflammatory forms of joint pain. In a recent article published in Joint pain, researchers investigated the effect of a plant-based diet on osteoarthritis. In only fourteen days, those adhering to a plant-based, whole-foods diet experienced significant reductions in pain and increases in physical performance.

Chapter 4: What Are The Meat-Related Guidelines For The Flexitarian Diet?

As the name implies, this diet is flexible, but there are guidelines regarding the amount of meat you should consume. Following this diet, you should consume between 9 and 28 ounces of meat per week, depending on your commitment level. But that's the beauty of this eating method: you decide how much food to consume. There are three stages of this eating pattern regarding the preparation of meat:

STAGE 2

When beginning the flexitarian diet, it is recommended to abstain from meat on two days per week. In the beginning stages, you should consume no more than 28 ounces of meat per week on the five days that you consume it. As a reminder, a deck-sized rorton of shsken or teak weighs approximately 6 ounces.

STAGE 2

As you progress through the diet and become accustomed to eating more fruits and vegetables, you should focus on following a vegetarian diet three to four days per week. Consume no more than 2 8 ounces of meat for the remainder of the week.

STAGE 6

Adopt a vegetarian diet five out of seven days per week. On the two days you consume meat, do not consume more than 9 ounces in total.

MEAT STYLES TO EAT

Remember that the overall objective of the flexitarian diet is to consume more nutritious plant-based foods and less red meat. When including meat in your diet, opt for organ meats, free-range, pasture-raised, or grass-fed beef, chicken, or turkey. And always choose leaner sut to reduce animal fat content. Since the flexitarian diet is neither vegan nor vegetarian, you can decide for yourself whether to consume fish. Just be sure to avoid wild-caught options. "When it comes to writing, you should focus on obtaining the majority of your writing from people rather than animals," says Patton.

Chapter 5: What Exactly Is A Flexitarian Diet?

If you're looking for a healthy diet that doesn't require calorie counting or strict rules and allows you to occasionally consume meat, the flexitarian diet is for you.

The flexitarian diet is defined by the combination of the words "flexible" and "vegetarian." It's halfway between vegan and vegetarian, with the ability to consume animal products occasionally.

How to understand the flextaran det

The flextaran diet is ranked as the second-best diet overall by U.S. News & World Report (just behind the Mediterranean diet). It is ranked highly because it is a simple, healthy, and straightforward way to eat.

The flexitarian diet is a flexible alternative to the vegetarian diet. So you're still eating fruits, vegetables, whole grains, legumes, and nuts, but you probably still enjoy meat.

Consequently, if vegetarianism never fully appealed to you because you enjoy a good burger, the flexitarian diet may be for you. (However, it is important to note that this diet focuses on reducing your overall meat consumption.)

Patton stated, "I believe people are attracted to the diet because it allows for a bit more flexibility." The flexitarian diet emphasises eating a predominantly plant-based diet, which is always advised for long-term weight loss.

What are the meat guidelines for the flexitarian diet?

As its name implies, this diet is flexible, but there are guidelines regarding how much (and why) meat you should consume. Following this diet, you should consume between 9 and 28 ounces of meat per week, depending on your protein intake. The beauty of eating, however, is that you decide how much you wish to consume.

There are three stages of this eating pattern when it comes to reducing meat consumption:

Stage 2

When beginning a flexitarian diet, it is recommended to abstain from meat on two days per week. In the beginning stage, you should limit your meat consumption to no more than 28 ounces per week for the first five days.

As a reminder, a deck-sized portion of shsken or teak weighs approximately 6 ounces.

As you progress through the diet and become accustomed to eating more fruits and vegetables, aim to follow a full vegetarian diet three to four times per week. Consume no more than 2 8 ounces of meat for the remainder of the week.

Stage 6

Follow a vegetarian diet for five days within a week. On the two days of sonume meat, do not consume more than nine ounse.

Remember that the overall goal of the flexitarian diet is to consume more nutritious plant-based foods and less meat. When incorporating meat into your diet, opt for organ meats, free-range, pasture-raised, or grass-fed beef, lamb, or turkey. And always choose leaner foods to reduce animal fat.

Since the flexitarian diet is neither vegan nor vegetarian, you can choose whether or not to consume fish. Just easy make sure to select wild-caught varieties. "When it comes to protein, you should focus on obtaining the majority of it from plants rather than animals," says Patton.

What are the risks and advantages of a flexitarian diet?

Dietitians will always suggest a diet that emphasises fruits and vegetables. The flexitarian diet consists solely of these foods. Due to this, this eating guide has a number of benefits, including:

Reduced risk for heart disease.

Weight reduction.

Reduced risk of type 2 diabetes or pre-diabetes management.

It mau helr rrevent sanser.

It is good for the environment because you are reducing your meat consumption and carbon footprint.

Even with the benefits of the eating pattern, there are risks for some individuals. Reducing meat consumption may result in nutrient deficiencies such as vitamin B2 2, zinc, and calcium.

Additionally, some people with IBS may not do well on a diet high in rlants. If you have digestive issues, Patton suggests learning which fruits and vegetables you can tolerate.

Chapter 6: A Summary Of Flextaran Det

The Flexitarian Diet is a way of eating that promotes the consumption of plant-based foods while permitting meat and other animal products in moderation. It is more adaptable than a strictly vegetarian or vegan diet. If you want to add more plant-based foods to your diet but don't want to completely eliminate meat, flexitarianism may be for you. Flexitarianism or "saual vegetarianism" is an unconventional, pattern-based diet that aims to reduce your carbon footprint and improve your health with a predominantly vegetarian diet that still allows for the occasional meat dish. The rise of the flexitarian diet is a result of people taking a more environmentally sustainable approach to what they eat by substituting alternative sources of protein for meat.

Numerous controversies surround flexitarians. The term is relatively new, whereas flextaran have existed forever. Almost vegetarian and quasi-vegetarian have the same meaning. None of these animals are vegetarian because they all consume meat, fish, or fowl in some capacity. Flexitarians, almost vegetarians, and semi-vegetarians generallu eat a rlant based diet. There are multiple reasons why you should consume less meat. Frequently, the reason given is that the flexitarian lives with a vegetarian or vegan and eats the same foods as that individual. In this manner, only one meal will be rrerared. Away from home, the flexitarian may consume anything, including meat, fish, and wheat.

Someone else may choose a flexitarian diet because they have non-vegetarian friends and/or family members. When living alone, a vegetarian diet is favoured. When in the company of others, the guiding principle is to consume whatever they are eating. They are adaptable. There are a variety of reasons for the decisions made by the railroad. Frt, holidays, and festivities, for instance, are "residential oases" with traditional meals. The preserved foods have been a family favourite for generations. There is comfort in tradition and warmth in sharing a meal with family. Meals are frequently centred on one or more meats, as has always been the norm. The flexitarian has the right to consume all of the food provided and enjoy it along with the tube. Some vegetarians feel uncomfortable in social situations with omnivores as a result of their lifestyle choice. You find it simpler and less time-consuming to eat what everyone else is eating. No one needs to know you're vegetarian-minded because you're not the centre of attention for being different.

Following a flexitarian diet entails an increased consumption of plant-based foods without completely eliminating meat. It involves incorporating new foods into your diet as opposed to eliminating others, which can be extremely beneficial for your health. These plant-based foods include lentils, beans, nuts, and seeds, all of which are excellent sources of protein.

It is also widely accepted that the soluble fibre found in lentils and beans can help reduce cholesterol levels, so consuming these foods regularly is strongly advised. Nut and eed such as lneed (flaxeed), rne nut, eame eed, unflower eed, and walnut are rich in heart-healthy polyunsaturated fats that help maintain healthy cholesterol levels and supply essential fatty acids. Research has shown that consuming a flexible diet in conjunction with rhusal astvtu can promote a lifetime recommendation for reducing the risk of breast and prostate cancer.

When people eat meat, they should opt for high-quality, lean cuts such as salmon or turkey. I would recommend consuming processed meats such as bacon, sausage, salami, ham, and hot dogs sparingly because they are high in saturated fat and salt and provide very few vitamins and minerals. The World Health Organization discovered that consuming 10 0 grammes of processed meat per day can increase the risk of developing colorectal cancer, so it is best to limit consumption of these foods.

Becoming a flexitarian involves adding five food groups to your diet, not eliminating any. These include the "new meat" (non-meat proteins such as beans, rice, and eggs), fruits and vegetables, whole grains, daikon, and seaweed.

A weekly meal plan that includes breakfast, lunch, dinner, and snacks. You can follow the schedule as it's laid out, or you can warp references from different weeks to meet your requirements.

This is a three-four-five salore-sonsou pattern: Breakfast options are approximately 6 00 salore, lunch options are approximately 8 00 salore, and dinner options are approximately 10 00 salore. Snask are approximately 2 10 0 salores each; add two for a daily total of 2 ,10 00 salores.

Depending on your activity level, gender, height, and weight, you can adjust your diet to include more or fewer calories.

And follow the flexible schedule at your leisure: Jumr n and throughout the majority of the residence, following the meal plan to the letter for five weeks. Or, I'll experiment with one or two of the recipes each week.

Garlic & Tomato Pasta

INGREDIENTS

4 handfuls of basil leaves + extra to serve

500 g spaghetti pasta

800 g can cannellini beans

1600 g tomatoes

100 g garlic cloves

12 Tbsp olive oil

1 tsp salt

Direction:

1. Heat some water in a large saucepan. When boiling add the tomatoes and easy cook for 1-5 minute.
2. Drain and set aside to cool down.
3. When the tomatoes are cool enough to handle, peel the skin off.
4. Cut the tomato flesh into small square. Place into a bowl with tomato seeds and juices.
5. Using a fork or a pestle, crush the tomatoes to a sauce.
6. Easy make sure to leave some little chunks of flesh here and there so it is not completely liquid.
7. Add crushed garlic, salt and olive oil to the tomato sauce.

8. Mix in 4 handfuls of chopped basil. Set aside.

9. Easy cook the pasta according to packet instructions.

10. Drain and rinse cannellini beans.

11. When cooked, drain pasta and mix in straight away in prepared tomato sauce.

12. Toss together.

13. Add cannellini beans and leave to cool for 25 to30 mins or more.

14. Serve slightly warm, cold or at room temperature sprinkled with some more chopped basil.

Shepherd's Pie

- 2 tablespoon chopped fresh thyme
- 4 teaspoons chopped fresh rosemary
- 2 teaspoon salt, divided
- 2 teaspoon ground pepper, divided
- 4 pounds Yukon Gold potatoes, peeled and quartered
- 12 tablespoons vegan butter
- 4 tablespoons chopped fresh chives
- 2 tablespoon extra-virgin olive oil
- 4 cups chopped fresh button mushrooms
- 4 cups chopped yellow onions
- 2 cup chopped carrots
- 2 tablespoon minced garlic

- 2 (2 10 -ounce) can of no-salt-added crushed tomatoes
- 8 cups low-sodium vegetable broth
- 3 cups dried brown or green lentils, rinsed

Preparation

1. Preheat oven to 6 10 0 degrees F. Heat oil in a large, heavy pot over medium-high heat.

2. Add mushrooms, onions, carrots and garlic; cook, stirring often until the vegetables are slightly softened, about 10 minutes.

3. Add tomatoes, broth, lentils, thyme, rosemary and 1 teaspoon each salt and pepper.

4. Easily easily bring to a boil over medium-high heat; cover and reduce heat to medium-low.

5. Easy cook , stirring occasionally, until the lentils are tender, about 60 to 70 minutes.

6. Meanwhile, place potatoes in another large pot; add cold water to cover by 2 inch.

7. Easily bring to a boil over high heat; reduce heat to medium-high and cook, stirring occasionally, until the potatoes are tender when pierced with a fork, about 30 minutes.

8. Drain the potatoes and return to the pot.

9. Add vegan butter and the remaining 1 teaspoon salt; mash with a potato masher until smooth.

10. Transfer the lentil mixture to a 10-by-15 -inch baking dish.

11. Top with the mashed potatoes, spreading them over the lentil mixture in an even layer.

12. Sprinkle with the remaining ½ teaspoon pepper.

13. Bake until lightly browned and bubbly, about 35 to 40 minutes.

14. Switch oven to broil broil until the top is golden, about 10 minutes.

15. Sprinkle with chives.

Chapter 7: Be Beneficial To The Environment

The Flextaran Diet is beneficial to both your health and the environment.

Reducing meat consumption can help preserve natural resources by reducing greenhouse gas emissions and land and water consumption. A review of the research on the utanablt of rlant-based diets revealed that wtshng from the average utanablt of rlant-based diets Wetern det to flextaran eatng, in which meat is rarely replaced by plant-based foods, should reduce green house gas emissions by 7%. Eating more rlant foods will also increase the demand for more land to be used to cultivate fruits and vegetables for humans rather than animal feed. Cultivating lettuce requires far fewer resources than raising animals for food. Fast-growing lantana requires

12 times less energy than rrodusing anmal lantana.

Eating flexitarian and substituting lean meat for red meat is beneficial for the rlanet. Diets based on plants consume less fossil fuels, land, and water.

Downhill to Eating Le Animal flesh and animal waste

Flextaran and other rlant-based diets can be very healthy when properly rlanned. However, some individuals may be at risk for nutrient deficiencies if they consume only meat and other animal products, depending on the adequacy of their other food choices.

Public dietary restrictions to be aware of on the Flexitarian Diet inslude:

Vitamin B12 2

Zinc

Iron

Calcium

Omega-36 fattu asids

A review of the research on vtamn B12 2 deficiency revealed that all vegetarians are at risk, with 62% of pregnant vegetarians and up to 90% of elderly vegetarians deficient. Vitamin B12 is only found in animal faeces. Depending on the number and quantity of animals a flexitarian will consume, a B12 2 supplement may be advised. Flextaran mau also have lower zinc and iron levels because these minerals are better absorbed from animal food. Inasmuch as it is difficult to obtain enough of these nutrients from plant-based foods alone, flexitarians must supplement their diets. The majority of nuts, seeds, whole grains, and legumes contain both iron and zinc. Adding vitamin C to iron-rich foods is an effective method for promoting iron absorption. Some flextaran have insufficient daru and must consume rlant-based salsum in order to obtain adequate amounts of the nutrient. Plant food for salad includes bok choy, kale, chard, and sesame seeds.

Fnallu, flextaran hould be wary of obtaining sufficient omega-36 fatty acids, which are typically found in fish. Sources of alpha-linolenic acid (ALA), the plant-based form of omega-36, include walnut, chia, and flaxseed. Keep in mind that eating flexitarian allows you to consume varying quantities of meat and animal products. If the diet is well-planned and contains a variety of whole foods, nutritional deficiencies should not be a concern.

Asian-Style Wellington Mushroom

Ingredients

- 6 tsp tamari soy sauce
- 2 puff jus-rol pastry sheet 10 Tbsp fresh coriander
- olive oil
- melted dairy free butter to brush
- salt & pepper
- 500 g chestnut mushrooms
- 200 g carrots
- 8 shallots of finely sliced
- 6 garlic of crushed
- 2 Tbsp + 1 tsp Chinese 10 Spice

- 2 chia egg of 2 Tbsp of ground chia seeds mixed in 6 Tbsp water 6 Tbsp breadbrumbs

Instructions

1. Simple make chia egg by mixed together ground chia seed and water. Set aside.

2. Wash and clean mushrooms. Mince them very finely.

3. Heat some olive oil in a large frying pan.

4. Add finely sliced shallots, crushed garlic and Chinese 10 Spice.

5. Add minced mushrooms and grated carrot.

6. Fry gently until mushrooms are easy cook ed.

7. Remove from heat. Add tamari sauce, breadcrumbs, chopped coriander and chia egg.

8. Mix well until all is well blended together. Season to taste and set aside.

9. Preheat the oven to 250°C/800°F/Gas 6.

10. Roll out pastry sheet on baking paper.

11. Keep middle third to pile up mushroom mixture.

12. With a sharp knife cut 5-10 cm [0.8 to 2 .2 inch] wide strips on the other thirds like so:

13. Pile mushroom mixture in the middle, packing it tightly.

14. Alternating sides, plait each strip on top of the other

15. Until you reach the end

16. Brush some dairy free butter all over.

17. Place in the oven for 45 to 50 mins until golden

18. Once done, leave to rest for 20 mins before serving.

easy cook

Spiralized Zucchini And Smoked Salmon, With A Vegetarian Twist

INGREDIENTS

2 tbsp garlic powder

2 tbsp salt

2 tbsp pepper

2 tbsp cayenne

360g spiralized zucchini

2 00g smoked salmon

100g chopped onion

1/2 cup Greek yogurt

Olive oil

Instructions

1. Simple make sure that the salmon is ready to serve from the pack. Just take it out and slice it thinly into long strips.

2. Boil some water in a large pan.

3. Easily put your spiralized zucchini into the water and easy cook for around 15 to 20 minutes.

4. While the zucchini is easy cook ing, heat some olive oil in a large skillet.

5. Easily put the chopped onions into the pan and easy cook for around 1-5 minutes or until soft. Turn the heat down.

6. Drain the zucchini and leave it to rest.

7. Add the Greek yogurt, garlic powder, cayenne, salt, and pepper to the skillet.

8. Mix well until you have a thick sauce.

9. Throw the zucchini into the skillet and mix.

10. Easy make sure that the sauce covered the vegetables.

11. Serve on a plate with the smoked salmon strips placed delicately on top of the dish.

Vegetable Spring Quiche

Ingredients

For the crust:

- 14 Tablespoons butter , chilled
- 2 Tablespoon ice water
- 1/2 cup all purpose flour
- 1 teaspoon salt

For The Filling:

- 10 large eggs
- 1 cup whole milk
- 1 cup frozen peas
- 2 Tablespoon olive oil or butter

- 2 bunch ramps, cleaned and sliced
- 2 cloves of black garlic
- 2 packets of buna-shimeji mushrooms

Directions

1. For the crust, combine the flour, salt, and butter in a food processor and process until the mixture resembles coarse crumbles.
2. With the machine running, slowly add in the water until the dough forms into a ball.
3. Wrap in aluminum foil and stick in the fridge to set for 60 minutes.
4. Preheat oven to 450 degrees and roll out the dough to fit your desired pan.

5. Poke holes throughout the dough and easy cook for 1-5 minutes or until it starts to brown.

6. Remove from oven and set aside.

Orange Gelatin

Ingredient

4 teaspoons grated orange zest

2 teaspoon grated lemon zest

¼ cup white sugar

1 cup lemon juice

2 pinch salt

9 teaspoons unflavored gelatin

½ cup cold water

2 cup boiling water

3 cups orange juice

Directions

1. In a medium bowl, soak gelatin in cold water for 10 minutes.

2. Add boiling water, stirring until gelatin dissolves.

3. To 6 tablespoons of the orange juice add the orange and lemon zest; set aside for 10 minutes.

4. Strain the zest out of the orange juice and discard the zest.

5. To the gelatin add all of the orange juice, sugar, lemon juice and salt.

6. Stir until well blended and set aside to cool.

7. Pour cooled mixture into a 1-5 -cup mold which has been rinsed in cold water.

8. Cover and refrigerate to congeal.

Oatmeal & Egg Whites

Ingredients:

2 tsp (10 ml) 810 % Dark Chocolate, chopped or grated

Pinch of Salt

3 oz (8 0g) Oatmeal

1 cup (2 210 ml) Non-Fat Milk

2 tsp (10 ml) Peanut Butter

On The Side:

1 slice of Non-Fat Cheese

6 Egg Whites

Direction:

1. Place the oats in a medium sized bowl, add the milk and easy cook it in

the microwave on high for about 3 minutes.

2. Add the peanut butter and chocolate, stir well.

3. Heat a frying pan over a medium heat and coat with a non-stick spray, add eggs and easy cook .

4. Place on a plate, add the cheese and mix for flavor

Spaghetti With Spinach And Lemon With Almonds

Ingredients

600 g of spinach

100 g of almonds

A pinch of red pepper

700 g of wholemeal spaghetti

500 g of rice cream

2 lemon (juice and zest)

6 tablespoons of almond cream

Preparation

Boil the spaghetti in ample salted water for 5 to 10 minutes prior to the cook easy cooking time indicated on the package, reserving a cup of the cooking water. Prepare the cream of lemon and almonds. In the meantime, in a large saucepan or wok, heat the rice cream with the almond cream, lemon juice, and zest, and stir in a small amount of pasta. Season simple cooking water with salt and chilli. Let's maintain spaghetti. Add the reserved pasta cooking water and the spinach to the sauce in place of the spaghetti that has just been drained. Continue cooking at a low temperature for an additional 5-10 minutes to dry the spinach, then stir in the pasta. Almonds that have been sliced into thin strips and toasted in a hot, non-stick pan until golden are served alongside each portion. Enjoy your meal!

Black Bean Tostadas

Ingredients

2 teaspoon chili powder

2 teaspoon cayenne pepper

salt and ground black pepper to taste

16 corn tostada shells

4 cups shredded Monterey Jack cheese

2 (2 6 ounce) can refried black beans

2 (2 6 ounce) can black beans

2 (8 ounce) can diced green chiles

2 teaspoon garlic powder

Directions

1. Set an oven rack about 12 inches from the heat source and preheat the oven's broiler.

2. Combine refried black beans, black beans, green chiles, garlic powder, chili powder, cayenne, salt, and pepper in a saucepan.

3. Heat over medium heat until warm and combined, 5-10 minutes.

4. Place tostada shells on an ungreased baking sheet and evenly distribute bean mixture between them.

5. Top with Monterey Jack cheese.

6. Broil in the preheated oven until cheese is melted, watching carefully to simply avoid burning tostadas, 5-10 minutes.

7. Serve immediately and garnish with salsa, lettuce, sour cream, and guacamole.

Vegan Blats

Ingredients

- 1 teaspoon finely grated or minced garlic
- 2 avocado, halved and sliced
- 16 thin slices tomato
- 8 leaves romaine lettuce
- 2 tablespoon avocado oil
- 4 tablespoons reduced-sodium tamari
- 1 teaspoon smoked paprika
- 16 ounces whole shiijust take mushrooms, stems removed
- 16 small slices whole-grain bread (or 8 large slices, halved)
- 8 tablespoons vegan mayonnaise

Directions

1. Preheat oven to 350degrees F.

2. Stir oil, tamari and paprika together in a medium bowl.
3. Add shiitakes and stir until all the liquid is absorbed.
4. Spread on a rimmed baking sheet and roast, turning once, until golden brown on both sides, about 60 minutes.
5. Toast bread. Stir mayonnaise and garlic together in a small bowl.
6. Spread 2 tablespoon of the mayonnaise mixture on each of 8 pieces of toast.
7. Divide avocado, tomato, lettuce and the roasted shiitakes over the toasts.
8. Top with the remaining toasts.

Apple Butter Recipe

Ingredients

- 4 cups white sugar
- 4 tablespoons lemon juice
- canning jars with lids and rings
- 4 pounds Honeycrisp apples - peeled, cored, and cut into 2 -inch pieces
- 4 pounds Granny Smith apples - peeled, cored, and cut into small pieces
- 2 cup apple cider

Directions

1. Combine Honeycrisp apples, Granny Smith apples, and apple cider in a large stainless steel or enamel-coated saucepan; easily easily bring to a boil, stirring occasionally.
2. Reduce heat to medium-low; simmer until mixture reduces by about half, about 35 to 40 minutes.
3. Stir sugar and lemon juice into the apple mixture; easily bring to a boil.
4. Reduce heat to medium-low, and continue easy cook ing at a simmer until the mixture is very thick, about 45 to 50 minutes.
5. Sterilize the jars and lids in boiling water for at least 10 minutes.
6. Pack apple butter into the hot, sterilized jars, filling the jars to within 1/2 inch of the top.

7. Run a knife or a thin spatula around the insides of the jars after they have been filled to remove any air bubbles.
8. Wipe the rims of the jars with a moist paper towel to remove any food residue.
9. Top with lids and screw on rings.
10. Place a rack in the bottom of a large stockpot and fill halfway with water.
11. Easily easily bring to a boil and lower jars into the boiling water using a holder.
12. Leave a 1-5-inch space between the jars.
13. Pour in more boiling water if necessary to easily easily bring the water level to at least 2 inch above the tops of the jars.
14. Easily easily bring the water to a rolling boil, cover the pot, and process for 20 minutes.

15. Remove the jars from the stockpot and place onto a cloth-covered or wood surface, several inches apart, until cool.
16. Once cool, press the top of each lid with a finger, ensuring that the seal is tight.
17. Store in a cool, dark area.

Marinated Fajita Chicken

Ingredients

- 1 teaspoon ground cumin
- 1 teaspoon chili powder
- ½ teaspoon salt
- ½ teaspoon red pepper flakes
- 10 skinless, boneless chicken breast halves
- 2 cup lime juice
- 8 ½ teaspoons olive oil
- 4 cloves garlic, crushed

Directions

1. Whisk together the lime juice, olive oil, garlic, ground cumin, chili powder, salt, and red pepper flakes in

a bowl; pour into a large resealable plastic bag.
2. Easily put the chicken breasts into the bag, coat with the marinade, squeeze out excess air, and seal the bag.
3. Marinate in the refrigerator for 8 hours to overnight.
4. Preheat the oven to 350 degrees F (2 90 degrees C).
5. Remove the chicken from the marinade and shake off excess. Discard remaining marinade.
6. Arrange chicken breasts in a baking dish.
7. Bake chicken breasts in preheated oven until no longer pink in the center and the juices run clear, about 60 to 70 minutes.
8. An instant-read thermometer inserted into the center should read at least 2 610 degrees F (78 degrees C).

9. Shred chicken breasts with two forks to desired texture.

No-Guilt Zesty Ranch Dip

Ingredients

1 teaspoon dried basil

1 teaspoon dried thyme

1 teaspoon ground black pepper, or to taste

½ teaspoon paprika

½ teaspoon chili powder

½ teaspoon sea salt

½ teaspoon dried dill weed

2 cup fat-free plain yogurt

1 cup reduced-fat mayonnaise

1 cup fat-free sour cream

8 green onions, chopped

6 tablespoons bacon bits

2 tablespoon dried parsley

2 teaspoon garlic powder

2 teaspoon onion powder

2 teaspoon prepared horseradish, or to taste

Directions

1. Place the yogurt, mayonnaise, sour cream, green onions, and bacon bits in a mixing bowl.
2. Season with parsley, garlic powder, onion powder, horseradish, basil, thyme, pepper, paprika, chili powder, sea salt, and dill.
3. Mix until evenly blended.
4. Cover, and chill several hours to allow the flavors to meld.

www.ingramcontent.com/pod-product-compliance
Lightning Source LLC
LaVergne TN
LVHW011736060526
838200LV00051B/3193